Healthy Aging For Men & Women

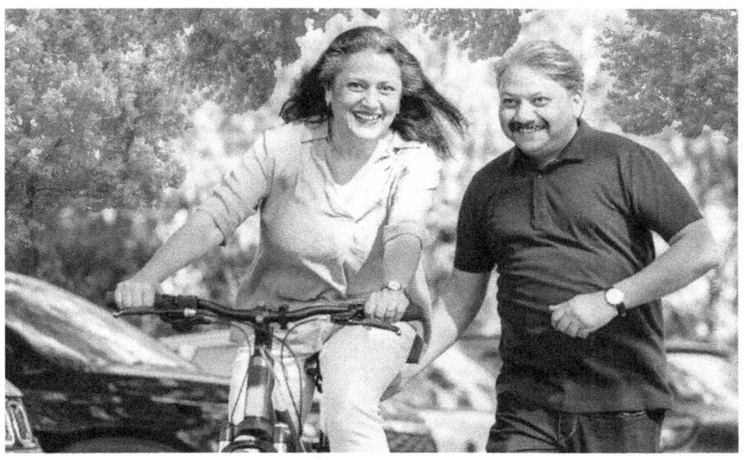

By: Debbie Pearl

TABLE OF CONTENTS:

CHAPTER 1. INTRODUCTION

Embracing the Journey of Healthy Aging

What exactly do we mean by "Healthy Aging"?
In order to preserve and enhance physical and mental health, independence, and quality of life throughout the course of a person's lifetime, healthy aging is a continual process.

Healthy aging is impacted by several variables. Some of them are beyond our control, including genetics. Others, including physical activity, a balanced diet, routine medical visits, and attention to our mental health, are within our grasp. You may take steps to manage your health, live as independently as possible, and preserve your quality of life as you age, according to research sponsored by NIA and others. Continue reading to find out more about the study and the actions you can take to encourage healthy aging.

At the biological level, aging is caused by the buildup of several types of cellular and molecular damage over time. As a result, physical and mental abilities gradually deteriorate, illness risk increases, and eventually, death occurs. These changes are not linear nor consistent, and they only tangentially correspond to an individual's age expressed in years. Age-related variety is not a coincidence.

Aside from biological changes, aging is often linked to other life transitions including retirement, moving to a more suitable home, and losing friends and companions.

Aging is a journey rather than a destination. It's a journey that plays out differently for all of us, filled with highs and lows, learning experiences, and treasured memories. The passing of time is a necessary aspect of life for both men and women, but how we handle it may make all the difference.

We set out on a transforming journey in this book that celebrates the grace of healthy aging in both men and women. It's a journey that goes beyond just existing and instead embraces life in all of its glory. Together, we'll examine the mental, emotional, and physical effects of becoming older and learn how to live longer and better lives.

As we go ahead, we will debunk prevalent fallacies about aging and swap them out with powerful realities. Through diet, exercise, and self-care, we'll discover how to promote physical vitality. We'll dive into the significant effects of mental and emotional wellness, realizing that they form the basis of a fulfilling existence.

This path is about accepting the grace and strength that come with each passing year rather than trying to achieve perpetual youth. It has to do with valuing the experiences that have left their marks on our faces, the laughter that still reverberates, and the aspirations that will continue to influence our future.

So let's start on this adventure together, whether you're in the prime of your life, close to a significant birthday, or enjoying the wisdom of your elderly years. Let's learn the keys to good aging, reexamine what it means to become older, and eagerly welcome life in all its richness.

Welcome to the path of healthy aging, where each day is a gift, each moment is an opportunity, and the best is yet to come.

What Happens To Our Bodies As We Age?

Certainly! Our bodies experience several alterations as we age. In plain and conversational language, here's how I'll explain it:

1. Skin: Because our skin ages, it becomes less elastic and prone to wrinkles. Apply sunscreen liberally!

2. Bones: They may deteriorate, which would make us more prone to fractures. Keep them robust with calcium and exercise.

3. Muscles: Typically, they weaken and diminish. Maintaining muscular mass may be aided by regular exercise.

4. Joints: Movement might be unpleasant due to the rising prevalence of arthritis. A healthy weight may be achieved by being active.

5. Heart: Blood vessels may stiffen up, raising the risk of heart disease. Keep your heart healthy by eating right and being active.

6. Lungs: During demanding tasks, it could become more difficult to breathe due to some capacity loss. Exercise regularly and give up smoking may help.

7. Eyes: When reading or looking at close-up items, vision might deteriorate. It's crucial to get the eyes examined from time to time.

8. Ears: Possible loss of hearing acuity. Hearing aids may be a huge assistance.

9. Brain: Cognitive processes like memory may alter. Solving puzzles or picking up new skills might help you stay cognitively busy.

10. Metabolism: Slowing down might result in weight gain. Manage this with a balanced diet and consistent exercise.

11. Immune System: You can become more vulnerable to infections as a result of it weakening. Your immune system may benefit from regular vaccinations and a nutritious diet.

12. Hormones: Menopause in women and decreased testosterone in males may both be caused by fluctuating hormone levels.

Always keep in mind that aging is a normal part of life and that although it has its obstacles, it also gives knowledge and new experiences.

CHAPTER 2. THE IMPORTANCE OF NUTRITION

As people age, nutrition becomes more important for both men and women's health. Let's look at the significance of diet for both sexes as they age:

1. **Bone Health:** Bones may weaken with advancing age. To keep bones healthy and lower the risk of fractures, it's essential to consume enough calcium and vitamin D. Given that women are more likely to develop osteoporosis, this is particularly crucial for them.

2. **Heart Health:** As people become older, both men and women run a higher risk of developing heart disease. In order to lower the risk of heart problems, a diet high in fruits, vegetables, whole grains, and lean meats may help control blood pressure and cholesterol levels.

3. Weight Management: With advancing years, maintaining a healthy weight becomes increasingly difficult. By supplying vital nutrients without adding extra calories, good nutrition may aid in weight management. Dietary balance and portion management are important.

4. Muscle Mass: With aging, muscle mass tends to decline, which may have an impact on strength and mobility. Maintaining muscle mass and function requires a sufficient protein intake as well as frequent strength-training workouts.

5. Changes in Hormones: Hormone levels change with age, particularly for women going through menopause. Intake of calcium and vitamin D should be increased to promote bone health during menopause as one strategy for managing these changes in diet.

6. Cognitive Health: Both men and women may lower their risk of age-related cognitive decline by eating nutrient-rich meals, such as those strong in antioxidants and omega-3 fatty acids, which can promote cognitive function.

7. Digestive Health: Digestive problems are not uncommon in older people. Constipation and digestion may both be aided by a diet high in fiber from fruits, vegetables, and whole grains.

8. Immune System Activity: A strong immune system requires a diet that is well-balanced and contains a range of nutrients. To aid in the defense against infections and diseases, this is crucial for both sexes.

9. Skin Health: Vitamins C and E may retain skin suppleness and lessen the effects of aging. Skin health is also influenced by proper hydration.

10. Mental and emotional health: A healthy diet may affect one's mood and mental state. Better mental health and general quality of life may both be influenced by a balanced diet.

11. Prevention of Chronic Illness: Age-related increases in the prevalence of chronic diseases including diabetes, hypertension, and certain malignancies may be prevented or managed with a healthy diet.

In conclusion, it is crucial for both men and women to maintain good nutrition as they age. It's a crucial component of general health and wellbeing. A balanced, nutrient-rich diet and a healthy lifestyle may help people have longer, more vibrant, and active lives as they age, even if the nutritional demands of men and women may differ somewhat. Individualized advice based on specific health and nutritional requirements may be obtained by speaking with a healthcare professional or certified dietitian.

Fueling Your Body for Optimal Health

Yes, without a doubt. Both men and women should nourish their bodies to maintain good health as they age. Let's have a brief and casual discussion about it:

Dietary balance: It's important to eat a variety of foods. Put a variety of vibrant fruits and vegetables, lean meat and fish, complete grains, and healthy fats on your plate. Your body will get the vital nutrients it needs from this.

Hydration: It's important to stay hydrated. Water promotes healthy digestion, blood flow, and general wellbeing. Get at least 8 glasses every day.

Placement Control: Keep portion quantities in mind. It's crucial to avoid overeating since as you age, your metabolism may slow down. Pay attention to your body's signs to hunger.

Sodium & vitamin D: Particularly as you age, these nutrients are essential for healthy bones. The best sources include fortified meals, leafy greens, and dairy products.

Protein: The health of your muscles depends on it. Maintain your muscle mass by eating lean meats, legumes, and nuts.

Fiber: Fiber promotes good weight management and assists with digestion. Foods rich in fiber include whole grains, legumes, and vegetables.

Limiting sugar intake and processed foods: Obesity and other health problems may result from consuming too much sugar. Try to limit your intake of processed meals and sugary snacks.

Positive fats: Choose the healthy fats that come from avocados, almonds, and olive oil. These fats boost the general well-being and the health of the brain.

Exercise routine: Maintaining flexibility, balance, and muscular strength requires continued physical activity. Even daily walks might have a major impact.

Sleep: For general health, getting enough sleep is crucial. Get 7-9 hours of good sleep each night.

Mental well-being: Your mental health should not be overlooked. Maintain relationships with loved ones, pursue interests, and reduce stress by relaxing.

Periodic Checkups: For routine examinations and screenings, see your healthcare practitioner. Early health concerns detection makes management simpler.

It's important to keep in mind that men and women may have somewhat different nutritional demands, so it's a good idea to speak with a medical expert or a registered dietitian to develop a tailored plan that meets your particular needs. You may age gracefully and have a healthier, more active life by following these recommendations.

CHAPTER 3. EXERCISE AND FITNESS

For general health and vitality, it's essential to maintain fitness as you become older.

1. The Value of Exercise as You Age

Physical Health: Numerous physical advantages may be obtained by regular exercise. It lowers the chance of developing chronic diseases including heart disease, diabetes, and osteoporosis, improves cardiovascular health, and helps people stay at a healthy weight.

Bone and Muscle Health: Bone density declines and muscle atrophy are two common effects of aging. Strength-training routines may assist maintain bone density and muscular mass.

■**Balance and adaptability:** Balance and flexibility become more crucial as you age for keeping your mobility and avoiding falls. These elements may be enhanced by practices like yoga and tai chi.

■**Mental Wellness:** The mental health benefits of exercise are significant. It may enhance cognitive performance, lower the risk of depression and anxiety, and elevate mood by generating endorphins.

■**Longevity:** According to studies, exercising often is linked to living a longer, healthier life. It may lengthen life expectancy and improve quality of life as people age.

2. Exercise Types:

Aerobic Exercise: Exercises that raise your heart rate and strengthen your cardiovascular system include walking, swimming, cycling, and dancing.

Set 150 minutes or more per week of moderate-intensity aerobic activity.

Strength training: Muscle mass may be built and maintained by lifting weights or utilizing resistance bands. Targeting main muscle groups, strength training should be done at least twice per week.

Balance and Flexibility Exercises: Your mobility will improve and your risk of falling will decrease if you include balancing training and stretches into your regimen. Excellent choices include tai chi and yoga.

3. Establishing a Workout Schedule:

Speak with a Healthcare Professional: Consult with your healthcare physician to be sure a new fitness program is safe and suitable for your specific requirements before beginning, particularly if you have underlying medical concerns.

Set Realistic Goals: Create fitness objectives that you can achieve and that are appropriate for your fitness level and age. This may keep you inspired and allow you to monitor your development.

Variety is essential: To avoid boredom and to train a variety of muscle areas, vary your routines. To keep things interesting, experiment with various workout forms.

Remain Hydrated: When exercising, proper hydration is essential, particularly as you become older. Prior to, during, and after your exercises, drink water.

Warm-up and cool-down exercises: To avoid injuries and lessen pain, always begin with a warm-up and conclude with a cool-down.

4. Maintaining Activity in Daily Life:

Include physical exercise: Seize every chance to move during the day. Take the stairs, walk instead of driving for short distances, and participate in physical activity-based hobbies.

Continue your social life: You may keep socially active and be motivated by participating in group activities or courses. A great approach to keep active and meet new people is to join fitness courses or clubs.

5. Listen to your body:

Pay rapt attention to the signs your body gives. It's important to treat any pain or discomfort you may feel when exercising, and seeing a medical expert or physical therapist may be helpful.

6. Retain a Positive Attitude:

A optimistic outlook may serve as a strong motivator. Celebrate your accomplishments and have a feeling of pride in your development to stay motivated.

7. Continual Checkups:

Routine check-ups may aid in maintaining your health and ensuring that any problems are dealt with as soon as they arise. Your healthcare practitioner should be informed about your workout program.

Remember that maintaining strength and mobility as you age is a lifetime endeavor. It's never too late to start, and even little adjustments may result in considerable improvements to your general health and standard of living. Customize your workouts to meet your interests and skills, and don't be afraid to ask for advice from healthcare practitioners or fitness experts to create a secure and efficient fitness program.

Best Exercises Suitable For Aged Men And Women

The best workouts for older men and women are listed here. While being easy on the joints, the following exercises may assist increase strength, flexibility, and general fitness:

1. Walking:

- One of the finest workouts for individuals of all ages is walking. It is simple to perform, low-impact, and adaptable to different fitness levels.

- To enhance cardiovascular health and general fitness, aim for brisk walking for at least 30 minutes most days of the week.

2. Swimming or water exercise:

- Water workouts provide resistance for muscular training while being easy on the joints.

- Swimming or doing water aerobics lessons may increase strength, flexibility, and cardiovascular fitness.

3. Chair Squats:

- This exercise works the quadriceps and other leg muscles in particular.

- Place a strong chair in front of you, sit down, and then without using your hands, stand back up. For 10 to 15 repetitions, repeat this motion.

4. Seated Leg Lifts:

- Place one leg straight out in front of you while sitting on a firm chair, hold for a few seconds, and then drop it back down. Repeat on the other leg. This exercise helps with balance and quadriceps strength.

5. Wall Push-Ups:

- From a standing position, lean in and execute a push-up against the wall with your hands at shoulder height on the wall.

- Push-ups against a wall bolster the triceps, shoulders, and chest.

6. Leg Extensions:

- Place your feet firmly on the ground while sitting in a chair. One leg should be raised straight in front of you, held for a brief period of time, and then brought back down. You may do this quadriceps-targeting exercise with or without ankle weights.

7. Arm Circles:

- Extend your arms out to the sides while standing or sitting. Make little circles with your arms and then progressively enlarge them.

- Arm movements develop the deltoid muscles and enhance shoulder mobility.

8. Tai Chi:

- Tai Chi is a slow-moving, low-impact martial art that encourages flexibility, balance, and mental calm.

- It works wonders for enhancing joint health and lowering the danger of falling.

9. Yoga:

- Yoga offers a range of stretches and positions that help improve balance and flexibility. It also has advantages for stress reduction and mental relaxation.

10. Resistance Band Exercises:

- Resistance bands are useful equipment for building strength. They are suitable for activities like seated rows, leg lifts, and bicep curls.

- You can change the amount of resistance with these, and they are easy on the joints.

It's crucial to speak with a healthcare professional before beginning any workout regimen, particularly if you have underlying medical issues. They can advise you on safe workouts that are appropriate for your particular requirements. To guarantee perfect form and technique for these workouts, you could also think about seeing a physical therapist or fitness expert.

CHAPTER 4. PREVENTIVE HEALTH MEASURES

Screening And Vaccinations For A Longer, Healthier Life

Let's go into further detail about the significance of screenings and immunizations for encouraging a longer, healthier life in older men and women:

Screenings:

1. Mammograms for women as part of cancer screenings Breast cancer detection relies heavily on mammograms. Around the age of 40, or as advised by their healthcare physician, women should begin routine mamammograms1.QMen's Prostate Cancer Screenings: Prostate cancer screening methods include digital rectal examinations (DRE) and prostate-specific antigen (PSA) assays. Men should talk to their doctor about screening's advantages and disadvantages, often beginning around age 50.

2. Colonoscopy: Both sexes need to have routine colonoscopies to screen for colorectal cancer. Depending on personal risk factors, this usually begins from 45 to 50 years of age.

3. Blood Pressure: Monitoring blood pressure is crucial since it may cause heart disease and stroke. Early adulthood should mark the start of routine examinations that last throughout life.

4. Cholesterol Levels: Heart disease is influenced by high cholesterol. Regular testing aids in identifying increased cholesterol levels, enabling early management via dietary adjustments or medication.

5. Bone Density Testing: Bone density scans, or DEXA, are essential for women, particularly after menopause, when the risk of osteoporosis rises.

These scans determine the fracture risk and the state of the bones.

6. Diabetes Screening: Blood sugar testing, such as fasting glucose or A1C tests, can diagnose diabetes or prediabetes. Early detection enables lifestyle adjustments and prompt medical care.

Vaccinations:

1. Influenza Vaccine: Older persons are more vulnerable to serious flu complications, thus being vaccinated against the flu each year is strongly advised. It lowers the likelihood of becoming unwell and needing hospitalization.

2. Pneumococcal vaccine: Pneumonia in elderly persons may be quite serious. For people 65 and older, or earlier for those with certain risk factors, the pneumococcal vaccination is administered in two versions (PCV13 and PPSV23).

3. Shingles Vaccine (Herpes Zoster): The shingles vaccine is essential for persons over 50. The vaccination may lessen the risk and severity of the illness, which can cause highly painful shingles.

4. Booster injections are required to maintain immunity for tetanus and pertussis (whooping cough), also known as Tdap. For individuals who interact with newborns, they are extremely crucial.

5. The HPV vaccination is not just for teenagers. Adults up to the age of 45 are advised to get it, particularly if they didn't have it when they were younger since it can protect against several malignancies.

6. COVID-19 Vaccine: The continuous fight against the virus depends on COVID-19 vaccinations. They guard against serious sickness and assist in slowing its spread. Additionally, booster injections could be advised for elderly persons.

Screenings and vaccines are preventative procedures that can have a big influence on how long and how well older men and women live. It's essential to have regular conversations with medical professionals to decide on the right screening schedule and immunization regimen depending on age, risk factors, and personal health histories. The key to living a longer, healthier life in one's older years is to take these preventative steps.

CHAPTER 5. SOCIAL CONNECTIONS

The Strength of Social Networks in Healthy Aging

Think of a world without loved ones, friends, or the reassuring chats that make you smile. Especially as you get older, it's not a world you'd want to live in. Social interactions, as it turns out, are kind of like the key to good aging. Let's investigate why.

1. The Fountain of Youth

Ever notice how spending time with family and friends may make you feel younger? It's science, not simply a sensation, after all! Strong social ties may, according to studies, really slow down the aging process.

2. A Sound Heart

The human heart craves company. Strong social bonds are associated with healthier hearts in individuals. Your heart beats more steadily when you converse, laugh, or exchange tales, which lowers your chance of developing heart disease.

3. Sharper Minds

Making new friends is a mental exercise. You may keep your mind active and stave off cognitive loss as you age by participating in stimulating discussions, activities, or even friendly disputes.

4. Emotional Adaptability

Curveballs are thrown by life, but having a support network makes it simpler to manage. Your ability to cope with stress, anxiety, and even depression is improved when you have friends or family to draw on.

5. Persistence in Exercise

People you know may serve as your workout partners. Maintaining an active lifestyle is more enjoyable and holds you responsible when you go for a walk with a buddy or enroll in a group exercise class.

6. Living with a purpose

Relationships give one a feeling of direction. Your relationships give your life significance, whether it's taking care of your grandkids, giving back to the community, or just being there for loved ones.

7. An Immunity Boost

Having friends, it's true, helps boost your immune system. Your body's ability to fight off ailments is strengthened by positive social connections.

8. Quality Over Quantity

Having deep connections is more important than having a ton of pals. Your wellbeing may be greatly improved by even a small number of intimate relationships.

9. The best medicine is laughter

Laughter with friends is a great stress reliever. It elevates your mood by releasing endorphins, the feel-good chemicals in your brain.

10. The capacity to adapt to change

As life changes, so do the adjustments, and having social ties helps. Your support network aids in your ability to adjust to new situations, such as retirement, the death of a loved one, or relocation.

11. One's Lifelong Journey

Making social relationships isn't only for kids. All throughout your life, they are essential, and as you get older, their value increases. So, treat your relationships like the rare jewels they are by taking care of them.

In a word, your connections are like a gold mine of wellbeing. So, get in touch with a buddy, spend time with relatives, or establish new relationships. If you embrace the power of social relationships, you'll discover that growing older can be a fulfilling and happy journey with the people you love by your side.

CHAPTER 6. FINANCIAL PLANNING

Securing Your Future And Peace of Mind

Visualize this, you're on a trip, and the map you're following will take you there. That map is similar to financial planning; it aids you in navigating the financial bends and turns of life so that you may achieve your objectives and find peace of mind.

1. Setting Clearly Defined Goals:

Financial planning begins with establishing certain objectives. What do you want to accomplish in the near future like a vacation or the far future like retirement? You may map out your financial course with the support of your ambitions.

2. Planning a budget:

Your spending strategy is outlined in a budget. It reveals your income and expenditures in terms of money. Making and following a budget is similar to having a sign that directs you in the right direction.

3. Disaster Relief Fund:

Life is full of unexpected events, not all of them good. An emergency fund may be used in this situation. It acts as a safety net, making sure you are equipped to handle unforeseen costs.

4. Planning for the Future:

Saving money is essential for a variety of goals, including retirement, property ownership, and kid education. As though you were funding your "future happiness" account. You'll have more when you need it if you start early.

5. Taking care of debt:

Debt may be a difficult burden. Managing and lowering debt to prevent it from impeding your progress toward your objectives is a crucial component of financial planning.

6. Making Smart Investments:

Investing is like to sowing financial future-oriented seeds. It's about using stocks, bonds, or other investments to make your money work for you. Your wealth may increase with time thanks to it.

7. Insurance:

Insurance is your defense against the storms of life. When unplanned occurrences happen, your financial security may be protected by life, health, house, and vehicle insurance.

8. Planning for Retirement:

Picture retirement planning like preparation for a dream vacation. A pleasant retirement when the time comes is ensured by making contributions to retirement plans like a 401(k) or IRA.

9. Review and Modify:

Review your financial strategy on a frequent basis, just as you would while driving and reviewing your map. Your strategy needs to alter as life does.

10. Consult a professional for advice:

On occasion, you need a financial "tour guide." A licensed financial planner may provide professional guidance and assist you in developing a customized strategy.

11. Mental tranquility:

Finding peace of mind is ultimately what financial planning is all about. Knowing that you have a plan for the future, can accomplish your objectives, and are ready for life's ups and downs.

Do not forget that the goal of financial planning is to provide you the freedom to live the life you choose, not to limit it. It's about overcoming financial hardship and taking pleasure in the road while knowing that your future is safe. Start your financial planning journey now, and you'll see how it gives you confidence in the future and peace of mind.

Conclusion: Embracing the Journey of Healthy Aging

Our ability to negotiate the final chapters of life with grace, energy, and wisdom depends on our ability to embrace the path of healthy aging. This experience is transformational and uplifting. Let's come to some thorough conclusions about this voyage as we think back on it to capture its essence:

Age is a Privilege, Not a Burden: Healthy aging serves as a reminder that for many people, getting older is not a luxury. It's a special chance to appreciate the variety of life's events, to embrace the present, and to develop personally.

Health is Wealth: The quality of our aging journey is constructed on the basis of our health. We make a financial investment in the length and quality of our years by placing a high priority on physical fitness, a healthy diet, and yearly physical exams.

Mind Matters: Maintaining our mental health is just as crucial as looking after our physical health. Our brains remain flexible and robust thanks to ongoing learning, social interaction, and curiosity.

Social ties are lifelines: One cannot overestimate the importance of connections. Relationships with friends, family, and members of the community provide comfort, company, and a safety net at difficult times in life.

Life Is Fueled by Purpose: A feeling of purpose provides life direction and meaning. Finding contentment in one's career, hobbies, or volunteer activity gives each day a sense of direction and vigor.

Resilience in the face of adversity: Accepting healthy aging gives us the resiliency to overcome challenges with bravery and tenacity. It tells us that difficulties provide chances for development.

Celebration of Individuality: Every person's experience of becoming older is different. Let go of cultural constraints and concentrate on what makes us happy and fulfilled as we accept our uniqueness.

Making Plans for the Future: Planning for the future gives us peace of mind and security. It guarantees that we may enjoy our older years free from worry and financial uncertainties.

Adaptability is Important: Life is always changing, and our resilience is determined by how well we can adjust to these changes. Our aging journey is made more interesting by accepting change and keeping open to new experiences.

Gratitude Improves Quality of Life: The foundation of good aging is gratitude. When we give thanks, we enjoy the little things and see how beautiful each day is.

Finally, accepting the process of good aging is both an art and a science. It involves cultivating relationships and valuing the moments that make life remarkable while also taking care of one's health, mind, and soul. It demonstrates the tenacity of the human spirit and the fact that every era has its own distinct beauty and function. Let us go on this road with open hearts, accepting the grace and wisdom that come with the passage of time. In the end, it doesn't matter how many years you have left; what matters is how much life you have left.

www.ingramcontent.com/pod-product-compliance
Lightning Source LLC
Chambersburg PA
CBHW051713250726
48653CB00007B/3010